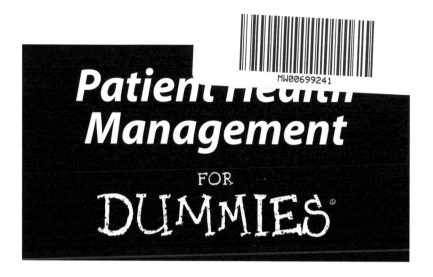

Patient Health Management

FOR DUMMIES®

by Dr. Terrence Montague

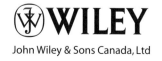

WILEY

John Wiley & Sons Canada, Ltd

Patient Health Management For Dummies®

Published by
John Wiley & Sons Canada, Ltd.
6045 Freemont Blvd.
Mississauga, ON L5R 4J3
www.wiley.com

Printed in Canada

1 2 3 4 5 TRI 08 07 06 05 04

Distributed in Canada by John Wiley & Sons Canada, Ltd.

For general information on John Wiley & Sons Canada, Ltd, including all books published by Wiley Publishing, Inc., please call our warehouse, Tel 1-800-567-4797. For reseller information, including discounts and premium sales, please call our sales department, Tel 416-646-7992. For press review copies, author interviews, or other publicity information, please contact our marketing department, Tel 416-646-4584, Fax 416-236-4448.

For authorization to photocopy items for corporate, personal, or educational use, please contact in writing The Canadian Copyright Licensing Agency (Access Copyright). For an Access Copyright license, visit www.accesscopyright.ca or call toll free, 1-800-893-5777.

About the Author

Dr. Terrence Montague is one of Canada's pre-eminent experts in disease management and health outcomes research. He is the author of *Patients First: Closing the Health Care Gap in Canada* and has published more than 300 academic papers and presentations.

Born in Saint John, New Brunswick, Dr. Montague graduated from Dalhousie University with a doctorate in Medicine. He is a vice-president at Merck Frosst Canada and leader of the patient health team.

Prior to joining Merck, Dr. Montague was Professor of Medicine and Director of Cardiology at the University of Alberta. He has occupied a number of academic positions at the University of Alberta, the University of British Columbia and Dalhousie University, and served on the editorial boards of the *Canadian Journal of Cardiology*, the *American Journal of Noninvasive Cardiology, Chest,* and *HealthCare Papers*.

Dr. Montague served with the Canadian Forces Medical Services in various roles in the Regular and Primary Reserve army in Canada and overseas. He retired with the rank of Lieutenant Colonel.

Author's Acknowledgements

I would like to thank Darryl Levine of Kelly+Aylen for his editorial and creative expertise, enthusiasm and dedication. I also thank John Aylen for sharing his invaluable wealth of publishing experience and judgment throughout the development process.

In addition I would like to thank the following people for their gracious comments and suggestions incorporated into the final content: from clinical and academic medicine and pharmacy, Drs. David Attwell and Ross Tsuyuki; from Merck Frosst Canada Ltd., Serge Labelle, Bonnie Cochrane, Joanna Nemis-White, Scott Wilson, Kurt Ryan, Trent Blackwell, Julie Hallé, Eileen Dorval, Elaine Andrews, Lori-Jean Manness and Michèle Beaulieu.

Any errors or omissions are mine alone.

Publisher's Acknowledgements

We're proud of this book; please send us your comments at canadapt@wiley.com. Some of the people who helped bring this book to market include the following:

Acquisitions, Editorial, and Media Development

Associate Editor: Robert Hickey

Manager, Custom Publications: Christiane Coté

Developmental and Copy Editor: Edna Barker

Project Manager: Liz McCurdy

Project Coordinator: Pamela Vokey

Cover Photos: Charles Thatcher/Getty Images

Production

Publishing Services Director: Karen Bryan

Publishing Services Manager: Ian Koo

Layout: Pat Loi

Proofreaders: Michelle Marchetti

Special Help

Darryl Levine

Publishing and Editorial for Consumer Dummies

Diane Graves Steele, Vice President and Publisher, Consumer Dummies

Joyce Pepple, Acquisitions Director, Consumer Dummies

Kristin A. Cocks, Product Development Director, Consumer Dummies

Michael Spring, Vice President and Publisher, Travel

Kelly Regan, Editorial Director, Travel

Publishing for Technology Dummies

Andy Cummings, Vice President and Publisher, Dummies Technology/General User

Composition Services

Gerry Fahey, Vice President of Production Services

Debbie Stailey, Director of Composition Services

Table of Contents

Introduction 1

Foolish Assumptions 1
What's in This Book 1
   Part I: Closing the Health Care Gap 2
   Part II: Launching a Patient Health
      Management Initiative 2
   Part III: The Merits of Measurement 2
   Part IV: Healthy Communication 2
   Part V: More than Ten Patient Health
      Management Initiatives 3
   Part VI: The Ten Major Themes in
      Patient Health Management 3
Icons used in this book 3

Part I: Closing the Health Care Gap 5

Understanding the Health Care Gap 6
Examining the Causes of the Health Care Gap 6
   Poor diagnosis 7
   Poor prescription 7
   Poor compliance 7
   Poor access 9
Closing the Care Gap with Patient Health Management 10
   Defining patient health management 10
   Looking at how a patient health
      management initiative works 11
   Exploring the characteristics of
      patient health management 13

**Part II: Launching a Patient Health Management
Initiative** 15

Getting Started 16
   Defining your initiative 16
   Determining scope 17
   Gathering the participants 17
   Allowing variation and thinking local 18
Creating a Steering Committee 19
   Composing the committee 20
      The executive champion group 20
      The writing team 21
   Understanding what a steering committee does 22

Part III: The Merits of Measurement 23

Understanding the Importance of Measurement 24
    Someone to watch over me: The Hawthorne effect ...24
    It's getting better all the time: The feedback loop 25
    You're number one: Focusing on patients 26
Making Measurement Count 27
    Building better data sheets 27
        Data sheet for initial visit 28
        Data sheet for follow-up visits 28
        How to design a data sheet 29
    Keeping people posted 29

Part IV: Healthy Communication 31

Educating Patients 31
    Kinds of education materials 33
    Patient-to-patient communication 33
Spreading the Word 33
    Sharing information with participants 34
        Newsletters and e-mails 35
        Meetings 35
    Keeping your peers posted 36

Part V: More than Ten Patient Health Management Initiatives 37

Part VI: The Ten Major Themes in Patient Health Management 41

Introduction

● ●

*T*his book has a simple message for health care professionals, patients, managers, governments and everyone interested in our health care system:

- ✔ Things can be better in our health care system.
- ✔ Care gaps exist in our health care system.
- ✔ Patient health management will close the care gaps and make things better by creating partnerships with all the players.
- ✔ Measurement and communication are key to making things better.

Foolish Assumptions

I have made a number of assumptions about you as a likely reader of this book. I assume

- ✔ You're a health care professional in Canada.
- ✔ You have an interest in population health research.
- ✔ You're curious about patient health management or disease management.
- ✔ You want to improve health outcomes for your patients or Canadians in general.

What's in This Book

This book is divided into six parts, with each part building on information contained in the previous ones.

Part 1: Closing the Health Care Gap

Every good book needs a hero and a villain. The villain is the care gap — the difference between best care and usual care. The hero is patient health management, a model for patient care that involves a community-based approach to treating patients at risk of disease. Bottom line: Patient health management works. Patient health improves.

In this part, I examine the four main causes of care gaps and how patient health management can help close care gaps.

Part 11: Launching a Patient Health Management Initiative

If you have a medical practice, you too can launch a patient health management initiative. More than a dozen successful programs have built a good knowledge base.

In Part II, I take you through the inner workings of patient health management, including the nitty-gritty issues like data collection, steering committees and communication.

Part 111: The Merits of Measurement

Rigorous measurement is a central element of patient health management and is integral to determining why and how medical therapies and practices work. Even the act of measuring appears to improve outcomes.

In Part III, I discuss the feedback loop and how repeated measurement and feedback generate continuous quality improvements in clinical and population health.

Part 1V: Healthy Communication

Communicating the results of your patient health management initiatives to health care professionals and patients will help generate interest and will stimulate thoughts and ideas to make things better.

In Part IV, I look at the best ways to communicate with your health care partners and patients.

Part V: More than Ten Patient Health Management Initiatives

This wouldn't be a ...For Dummies book if it didn't have a part of tens or two. In Part V, I describe twelve successful Canadian patient health management initiatives.

Part VI: The Ten Major Themes in Patient Health Management

I see several major recurring themes in successful patient health management, starting with the idea that things *can* be better and ending with the idea that things *will* be better. In Part VI, I summarize Montague's top ten themes of patient health management.

Icons used in this book

Peppered throughout the margins of the book are icons that flag important information. Here's a guide to what they mean.

This icon means the information is essential and you should be aware of it

This icon marks practical information you can use when you launch your patient health management initiative.

This icon is a red flag for you; it appears whenever I write about something you should watch out for.

Part I

Closing the Health Care Gap

* *

In This Part

▶ Defining the care gap

▶ Understanding what causes the care gap

▶ Defining patient health management

▶ Closing the care gap

* *

*I*n the early 1990s, I became the head of a major university cardiology research group. I was studying 2,079 heart attack patients who were being treated in hospitals in Canada. At the time we knew of three drugs that could prevent heart attacks. But less than half the people in the study were being treated with those drugs.

I was disappointed to discover that this problem was widespread — patients everywhere weren't getting the best possible care.

In this part, I look at the disparity between the best practices and the actual care patients receive, and I investigate what causes that gap. I also suggest a way to close it, a new model for patient care called patient health management. The goal of patient health management: the best health care for the most people at the best cost.

Understanding the Health Care Gap

The term *care gap* describes the differences between *best care* — therapy that's been proven to be effective, usually through large randomized controlled clinical trials — and *usual care* — the level of day-to-day care that patients actually receive. If we want to improve the health of patients, we need to find and close the care gaps.

Unfortunately, what we learn about best care is often not translated into action immediately. In the next section, we look at some of the reasons for this.

Examining the Causes of the Health Care Gap

We know that clinical studies and ongoing scientific research demonstrate the benefits of certain treatments, so why is there a care gap? Why aren't patients benefiting from the discovery of proven treatments? Answering this question is the first step to closing the care gap.

Researchers have identified the four top causes of care gaps:

- ✔ **Poor diagnosis:** The physician doesn't identify the patient's illness, or diagnoses the illness incorrectly.

- ✔ **Poor prescription:** The physician doesn't prescribe the most effective proven therapies or the correct dosing.

- ✔ **Poor compliance:** The patient doesn't follow the recommended treatment of drugs or lifestyle changes, such as diet and exercise.

- ✔ **Poor access:** The patient can't afford the recommended treatment or must wait to receive health services.

Who's responsible? Health care professionals, patients, governments and people who run public institutions, such as hospitals and clinics. But these people are also part of the solution. Everyone can help close the care gap.

Poor diagnosis

We don't have much data showing a causal link between poor diagnosis and poor outcomes, but plenty of anecdotal evidence can be found. Some diseases — particularly high blood pressure and osteoporosis — don't show symptoms for long periods, and these are the diseases that are most often mis-diagnosed. Until they *are* diagnosed, they can't be treated.

Poor prescription

Scientific knowledge is always growing, and scientists are always introducing new treatments. Yet, there's often a time lag before the more effective new treatments are commonly prescribed.

Several studies in Canada show that physicians often don't prescribe the most effective treatment for patients with life-threatening illnesses. For instance, a study of treatments given to patients admitted to hospital for heart attacks between 1987 and 1992 showed that less than half the patients received the proven drugs.

The care gap isn't limited to heart disease. The largest and most persistent care gap in diagnosis and prescription is in the field of osteoporosis. A multi-year survey and audit in Manitoba found that only about 20 percent of high-risk patients are optimally diagnosed and treated.

Poor compliance

The father of modern medicine, Sir William Osler, once said: "Man has an inborn craving for medicine." But Osler was only half right: data suggest that only half of us have this craving. Most patients stop taking their medication after only three to six months of therapy — even patients with chronic conditions like heart disease. Poor compliance costs Canada several billion dollars a year in reduced productivity. This is a significant lost opportunity for any society.

Being an active listener helps your patients

A friend of mine was having a hard time convincing his wife to take a life-saving medication prescribed by her physician. She refused to fill her prescription for a medication that was clinically proven to reduce her risk of stroke, heart attack or even death.

My friend tried to convince her with rational arguments about the clinical trial evidence. She refused. Then he appealed to her emotions by talking about losing quality of life and not being there for the kids. Still, she refused.

Finally, he asked the all-important question: "What is preventing you from taking this medication?"

She replied: "The idea of taking this drug for the rest of my life makes me feel old and I'm too young to feel old."

Prescribing physicians need to be active listeners so they can identify patients' concerns. Without dialogue, we have care gaps.

When doctors listen, patients can express their concerns. At the same time, doctors must provide professionally informed health information to the patient.

This way of communicating is called the *concordance model for patient-physician interaction*. It puts the patient first and at the centre of his or her health care.

Why do people stop taking their medicine? Studies suggest patients are influenced by

- Clinical settings, and their associated practices and processes
- Interactions between physician and patient in the care environment
- Severity of illness and complexity of treatment
- Cost and side effects of the therapy
- Availability of social support
- Knowledge of the disease and treatment alternatives, combined with a sense of *self-efficacy* (people's beliefs as to whether following the treatment will have a beneficial effect)

> ✔ Usual life routine and its likely degree of disruption by therapy
>
> ✔ Physician's ability to communicate the urgency of taking the medication and the risk of not taking it

Some research suggests that the more drugs a patient takes, the more likely the patient is to comply with the treatment.

Poor access

Studies show that the health of nations and the wealth of nations are connected. The healthier we are, the more well off is our society, and vice versa. In other words, our access to health care affects the degree to which we contribute to the economy, and the economy affects our access to the best treatment.

But institutional payers (our governments) often overlook this health-wealth relationship when they look for ways to meet short-term cost targets. The result: less access to health products and services leads to less-than-optimal health outcomes and reduced quality of life for patients. More people will require accute care and hospitalization, which will lead to ever higher government health care bills.

But here's the good news: In the future, care is likely to shift increasingly from hospitals to community settings as new and more effective therapies — particularly drug therapies — are administered in outpatient environments. Outcomes will improve and adverse effects will reduce the number of hospital admissions and readmissions.

Soon we should be able to provide better outcomes with less cost to the health system as a whole. For instance, clinical studies tell us that cholesterol-lowering drugs will improve the health of people with cardiac disease. The drugs may cause health expenses to increase in the short term. But making people healthy will reduce hospitalizations. Fewer people in hospitals will reduce hospital costs.

No country can afford to restrict access to innovative medical therapies if it aspires to be in the front rank of world health and economic outcomes.

Closing the Care Gap with Patient Health Management

Health care resources are often wasted because of the gap between knowledge gained from clinical trials and knowledge used to treat the community. Physicians may not prescribe the most effective drugs, and patients may not have access to them.

All patients want the best treatment possible. Imagine being told that simple treatment strategies exist to reduce health risks, but you're not receiving these treatments.

Canada will be a better, healthier and richer country if we can close the care gap. We need an accountable and feasible health management strategy that offers the best health for the most people at the best cost. Such a strategy exists. It's called patient health management.

Defining patient health management

Patient health management involves a community-based approach to treating patients at risk of a disease. The goal is to provide the best health for the most people at the best cost.

Patient health management initiatives typically involve partnerships between health care professionals (physicians, nurses, pharmacists), patient advocacy groups (Heart and Stroke Foundation, Osteoporosis Society and so on), private insurers, university professors, pharmaceutical companies and governments. Patients are the focal point of patient health programs.

Patient health management helps close the care gap by gathering and analyzing knowledge about what health care strategies and therapies work best — and ensuring the knowledge is passed on to those who can use it.

Patient health management addresses the four causes of the care gap and helps close the gap by

- ✔ Making health care professionals aware of the symptoms and diseases
- ✔ Providing health care professionals with the latest evidence-based clinical trial information
- ✔ Educating patients about their disease and the importance of taking their medications as directed
- ✔ Demonstrating the cost-saving benefits of clinically proven treatments to governments and other payers

Patient health management emphasizes partnerships, measurement and education to close the four care gaps — diagnosis, prescription, compliance and access. Patient health management works. Outcomes improve.

Looking at how a patient health management initiative works

In a typical initiative, health care professionals at local clinics and hospitals treat and track patients at risk of a disease. Data collectors compile and feed the data to the health care professionals who then act on the new evidence (everything you wanted to know about measurement but were afraid to ask is in Part III).

At the same time, physicians and others educate patients about their disease (I talk more about this in Part IV). Education tends to increase compliance with treatment and gives patients hope. Patients can take control and responsibility for their health care when they take their medications and make lifestyle changes.

Success in Nova Scotia

In 1997, a patient health management initiative was launched in Nova Scotia. Improving Cardiovascular Outcomes in Nova Scotia (ICONS) started as a five-year program that involved hundreds of health care professionals and thousands of patients across the province. The goal was to study and track heart health in Nova Scotia.

ICONS was not the first population-based study in Canada, but it was one of the largest. The program looked at patients hospitalized for heart disease at acute-care institutions in Nova Scotia and high-risk patients from physician practices across the province.

Cross-disciplinary clinical teams collaborated to make sure that patients received appropriate medication and advice about how to maintain their health. Treatment results were measured. Researchers monitored these results and gave the information to the clinicians to further improve patient care.

The result: patients took their life-saving medications, physicians received information on best practices and the Nova Scotia Department of Health reported an 18-percent reduction in the number of patients returning to hospital during the year following a heart attack.

Because of the very beneficial impact on the cardiovascular health of the population and the successful integration of community-based administrative culture and processes, ICONS became an operational program of the Department of Health of Nova Scotia in 2002. Policy-makers and health care administrators saw this successful patient health management initiative as a major innovation and achievement in organizational behaviour in primary health care.

ICONS markedly advanced techniques to enhance provider and patient communication, education and *buy-in*, that is, when stakeholders come to see the goals of the program as their own.

ICONS brought a culture of measurement to evidence-based practices and multidisciplinary health management. It enhanced interregional goodwill and sharing of best practices, and it laid the framework for a provincial cardiac program that became part of the day-to-day strategy and function of the Department of Health.

In short, ICONS demonstrated the success of the new partnership/measurement model for patient care: patient health management.

Exploring the characteristics of patient health management

Patient health management has eight characteristics (throughout this book I touch on a few):

- ✔ Patient-centred approach to prevention, diagnosis and management of illness

- ✔ Inclusion of drug and non-drug therapies

- ✔ Collaboration and coordination of services and interventions

- ✔ Focus on whole systems and not on isolated controls such as bed counts or hospital closures

- ✔ Monitoring, measurement and feedback of practices and outcomes

- ✔ System view of health and integration of components

- ✔ Improvement of the health of whole populations

- ✔ Knowledge creation and dissemination

Part II

Launching a Patient Health Management Initiative

· ·

In This Part

▶ Defining your initiative

▶ Bringing together the participants

▶ Creating a steering committee

· ·

I wonder if people in Caesar's Rome thought their health care was good and their life expectancy was long enough. Did they know that average life expectancy could be longer than 45 years? Did they know things could be better?

During the last half century the average life expectancy in Canada rose from about 68 to 80. This improvement did not occur by accident. Someone saw that things could be better and worked to make them better. Someone saw a gap and worked to close it.

Large care gaps can still be found in many of society's most burdensome illnesses. Things can always be better. Patient health management can help.

In this part, I explain how to launch a patient health management initiative in your clinic or community.

Getting Started

If you're like most health care professionals I know, your practice is full and you need ways to simplify administration — not add to it. And probably, like most health care professionals I know, you want to do whatever you can to help improve the health of your patients and your community.

The biggest fear about doing something new is making a mistake. Don't let fear keep you from doing *something*. The only real mistake is to do nothing.

An effective patient health management initiative requires three key components:

> ✔ **Data collection** — an accurate snapshot of what health care teams are doing
>
> ✔ **Data management** — health service consultants to help interpret the data and translate the findings
>
> ✔ **Committed stakeholders** — people whose goal is to ensure that individual patients have access to the best care at the best possible cost

Large patient health management initiatives can involve a region or an entire province and can include partnerships with national organizations, governments, pharmaceutical companies and universities. Smaller scale initiatives can track dozens of patients in a clinic or a few patients in one medical practice. The principles are the same.

Defining your initiative

Your location and patient group will help you decide the disease and the community you want to target in your initiative. Are you a family physician working in a rural office? Do you work in a downtown clinic with 10 other physicians? Are you in charge of a hospital department? What care gap do you want to close? Is there a particular disease you want to look at?

There is no wrong choice when it comes to launching a patient health management initiative. Your actions will help patients. You will make a difference. You may inspire other physicians to launch initiatives.

Determining scope

You need to determine the start and end points of your initiative. Will you track patient health results for two years or for ten years? How many patients will you include? You may not be able to track every major disease and every patient in your practice. Set realistic limits so you can achieve your goal.

Gathering the participants

You will need recruits for your initiative. To make it a truly community-based initiative, include physicians, pharmacists, nurses and other community stakeholders.

In a smaller initiative, many of these participants will form the steering committee. (I discuss steering committees a little later in this chapter.)

As a first step, make a list of colleagues you want to include. You'll have an easier time finding health care professionals willing to take part in large urban centres. But you can recruit a team in a rural area — just remember to consider geographic obstacles (for example, travelling for steering committee meetings).

Speak to physicians, pharmacists and nurses — they may help you find innovative ways to overcome geography to make your initiative a success.

Community-based stakeholders, including physicians, pharmacists and patients, will almost certainly view your patient health management initiative as innovative because it provides them with an opportunity to contribute to the generation and dissemination of medical information that might lead to important medical decisions.

Untapped community resources

Trusted organizations and community health care professionals can help recruit patients. But their influence and benefits extend to other areas of patient health management.

For instance, one of the ICONS (see Part I) sub-study protocols originated from the ideas of a community pharmacist who practiced in a very small town in northeastern Nova Scotia. He suggested the design of a randomized clinical trial. His presentation to the steering committee was compelling, was accepted and ultimately carried out. In subsequent committee meetings and in meet-and-greet activities, I noticed how influential and respected this pharmacist was with other members of the initiative.

The pharmacist combined an understanding of the importance of population health science and local civic sensitivity. Such talents are often available in communities. The pharmacist was a tangible manifestation of the moral authority inherent in the community. It just needs tapping and perhaps some measurement to make it operational.

The health care professionals you invite may never have been asked to make such a contribution before. But they'll likely seize the opportunity to contribute. Your local community has everyone you need to launch and sustain a patient health management initiative.

You will need data collectors who can compile the results of dozens or even hundreds of patients. The principal costs incurred in a typical initiative are funding for the data collectors and the expense of steering committee meetings.

Finally, invite your patients to participate. Explain your goal: to improve community health in a measurable way.

Allowing variation and thinking local

You don't need to impose uniformity. Every intervention need not be applied in every local setting.

Patients trust members of their community

During the ICONS patient health management initiative in Nova Scotia (see Part I), I discovered that patients and their families enrolled in the program were actively involved because community and patient groups, such as the Heart and Stroke Foundation, were firmly behind the goals of ICONS. From the executive director to the thousands of volunteers, everyone told patients and families that ICONS was a worthwhile project and should be supported.

Participation was a matter of trust. Patients trusted and listened to people they knew and respected in their community. That's why you need to ensure that your patient health management initiative is community-grounded and includes individuals and institutions your patients trust.

Partnership does not mean only sponsorship or financial commitment. Partners can contribute in many ways to the success of a patient health management initiative. For example, in ICONS, Merck Frosst provided business savvy — this industry partner offered advice and guidance to help ensure meetings were well organized, productive, and objectives were achieved.

In the total-quality-management world, we often think of variation as a bad thing. But in patient health management, variation at the community level might be a good thing. What works for Chicoutimi may not work in Lethbridge.

When you have before and after measurements for each setting, you can evaluate any differences. Allow for regional variation and flexibility so you can broaden stakeholder buy-in.

Creating a Steering Committee

A steering committee is the core of a patient health management organization.

Composing the committee

In smaller initiatives, the committee might include a few physicians, pharmacists, a nurse clinician, a patient or patient advocacy group and a dietician or other health care professional.

In larger initiatives, the committee should be big enough to convey a sense of community authority — which helps buy-in by stakeholders — but not so big that it's ineffective. A larger initiative might include partners from universities and from private and public organizations.

Community partners are vital, but so is balance. You may need to balance the sense of community authority, buy-in and empowerment that comes from a large steering committee with the need to get things done. A large work team may drift. A large steering committee needs a strong leader. So, for efficiency, create an executive champion group. A writing team is also useful. I look at both groups next.

The executive champion group

The *executive champion group* is a small part of the larger steering committee. It provides consistent leadership and administrative oversight to achieve the strategic goals and day-to-day running of the project. You and the other leaders of the initiative should be part of the group.

The executive champion group

- ✔ Hires staff
- ✔ Arranges meetings
- ✔ Creates data forms
- ✔ Coordinates with the data centre
- ✔ Determines who will be on the writing team (which I talk about next)
- ✔ Handles other administrative tasks

Leadership matters

Leadership is an elusive concept and hard to define, even though we know its importance and we all think we know what it means. United States Army General H. Norman Schwarzkopf said leadership is "getting others to do something they would otherwise not do." Having a durable value system and being faithful to it were also important to the general.

Dr. Garner King, a former colleague, said that effective leaders picked the best person for the job, communicated a vision and provided all possible support and communication to help people attain the vision and mission.

Leadership skills are essential in the field of population health, particularly in a patient health management initiative. Forming a community-based partnership and keeping it focused over the long term isn't easy. When it comes to leadership, try to remember that in the small-things department, less is more. For instance, try to avoid telling your partners how to do mechanical tasks, such as collecting and reporting measurements. If one partner wants to e-mail collected results and another wants to use a fax machine, well, why not? Too much rigidity can frustrate the process. In small matters, the best approach to leadership is often flexibility.

The writing team

The writing team communicates the project rationale, methods and results. They'll be your initiative's voice, providing information to participants, the community and scientific meetings and journals. A typical team may have two or three writers.

If you don't have a lot of experience writing, ask an experienced peer for help or consult with a professional medical writer. He or she can help you with style, grammar and format, while retaining the intent and thrust of the original text.

Understanding what a steering committee does

The steering committee usually meets two to four times a year to manage the business of the project, assessing progress, setting goals and developing action plans.

During a meeting, the steering committee might discuss such topics as

- ✔ Study results
- ✔ Intervention development and implementation
- ✔ Issues of process
- ✔ Didactic or interactive scientific presentations
- ✔ Professional development topics

Part III

The Merits of Measurement

. . . .

In This Part

▶ Knowing the importance of measurement

▶ Checking out the Hawthorne effect

▶ Looking at measurement tools

. . . .

*T*hese days, randomized clinical trials are ubiquitous. But this is a relatively new phenomenon. Scientific proof that patient outcomes are better with one therapy instead of another only recently became commonplace.

I was a practicing heart specialist in the early 1980s when I became aware of clinical trials as a practical tool for guiding management of patients with heart attacks. In the late 1980s, I was a participating investigator in the first randomized clinical trial to prove that a specific medication prolonged the life of patients with heart failure.

I discovered through those experiences that rigorous measurement is integral to determining why and how medical therapies and practices work. Consequently, measurement is an important part of patient health management.

In this section we look at measuring, how it affects patients and what to do with all those numbers and facts once you've collected them.

Understanding the Importance of Measurement

I can't overstate the importance of measurement in patient health management. Without measurement, health care professionals cannot say with certainty whether their prescribed treatment is helping their patients at the individual level. And without measurement, there would be no evidence that best practices are actually the best at the population or medical practice level!

Measurements tell us what works and what doesn't. Patient health management initiative leaders feed the best-practice information back to physicians so they can better treat their patients.

Measurement benefits everyone in an initiative. Patients are more compliant when you can show them just how a treatment works. And measurement encourages partners to focus on outcomes, rather than politics and administration. Measurement provides you with the tools to motivate.

So, what are the quantifiable benefits of measurement? Well, in this section I discuss how the very act of measuring improves results, how measurement can lead to constant improvement and how measurement keeps health initiatives focused on the patient.

Someone to watch over me: The Hawthorne effect

If you've tried to lose weight, you know the importance of measurement. You lose more weight when you track your weight loss. Weight loss centres know this, and track your weight every week.

Knowing that you're being monitored affects the way you act.

This effect was first noticed in 1927 at the Hawthorne, Illinois plant of Western Electric Company. Harvard researchers conducted a series of experimental interventions designed to have an impact on productivity. The researchers discovered that any intervention they tried — such as adding more light or reducing light to the production floor — improved productivity. Why? Because the interventions reminded workers they were being observed.

The Hawthorne effect can be defined as the initial improvement in a process of production caused by the obtrusive observation of that process. If you know your weight is being monitored, you may skip the fast-food lunch and stick to your low-fat diet.

If patients and health care professionals know you're measuring health outcomes from evidence-based care during a patient health management initiative, those outcomes tend to improve.

It's getting better all the time: The feedback loop

Measurement lets you see whether your intervention is working. But measuring is only the first of seven steps in the process of continuous improvements, called the *feedback loop*:

1. Baseline measurement
2. Analysis
3. Feedback
4. Interventions
5. New measurement
6. New analysis
7. New feedback

Interventions, guided by repeated measurement and feedback, generate continuous quality improvements in clinical and population health.

Analysis and feedback help you and your colleagues identify care gaps. Next, you develop and implement interventions aimed at closing the identified care gap(s). Then you compare your new measurements to baseline measurements to assess the degree of your intervention's success.

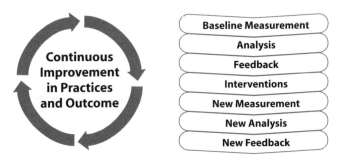

Figure 3-1: Repeated measurement and feedback generate continuous quality improvements in clinical and population health.

By continuously responding to ongoing feedback, we can have constant improvements.

Tracking and monitoring health care and results will improve health outcomes (the Hawthorne effect), and it also gives the health care professionals and administrators of the initiative useful information to continue improving patient health.

Sustaining the feedback loop is a challenge but an essential one if you want to maintain and enhance improved health outcomes. Without constant measurement and feedback, improvements may wane. If you integrate your measurement and feedback mechanisms into everyday practice, you'll ensure sustained quality improvement.

You're number one: Focusing on patients

The patient is the focal point of patient health programs. This may seem obvious, but I'm saying it anyhow — and I'll repeat it! Constant measurement and feedback improve outcomes. But measurement isn't enough. We also need to remind our patients and our community of our goal: improving patient health.

When we measure health data and communicate results to the community, we show whether we are getting the best return for our health dollars. Measurement can provide reassuring evidence to governments. Your partnerships with patient groups give payers and users of health resources reassuring evidence that their investment in health is improving outcomes.

Some governments understand the built-in fact-checking nature of patient health management and support patient health management initiatives. Such governments have chosen to manage the health care system not by cost alone; they also manage by outcomes.

As I have witnessed first-hand, when you manage by outcomes, you introduce the concept of evidence-based medicine. The patient becomes the focal point.

Making Measurement Count

Measuring data can be tricky business. Measurement can only happen if you solve the practical matter of tracking data effectively and accurately. Try to track too much information, and you may discourage your reporting health care professionals. Don't track enough, and you may end up with ambiguous or incomplete results.

Building better data sheets

A *data sheet* is a form that helps health care professionals track specific data points, such as date of visit, blood pressure, bone density results or whatever specific measurements are required to track the health change of a patient. It allows health care professionals to track accurate, precise and concise data for each project.

A bit of initial planning will give you a carefully designed, easy-to-use data sheet.

Every question on your form must pass the "why" test. Why is this information important? What do you need so you can track it? You need a very good reason for collecting information, and you must be satisfied that the information will provide value and contribute answers to the questions that generated the study. Ideally, a data sheet for any visit is never longer than one page.

Data sheet for initial visit

When the patient first visits, collect clinical and demographic information. Ask about the patient, the illness and any previous treatment and outcome. The first form might include:

- ✔ Patient's name or unique identifier
- ✔ Age
- ✔ Sex
- ✔ Social setting (for example, hospital, assisted living facility, at home and so on)
- ✔ Target disease diagnosis
- ✔ Relevant symptoms and physical signs
- ✔ Measure of severity (for example, frequency and degree of joint pain and degree of motion restriction in arthritis patients)
- ✔ Important family, concurrent or past illnesses
- ✔ Medications
- ✔ Allergies or side effects

Data sheet for follow-up visits

These information requests are usually shorter, and might include the following:

- ✔ Date of visit
- ✔ Any change in symptoms or severity
- ✔ Change in treatment regimens
- ✔ Hospitalizations since prior visit, and the cause
- ✔ Any other significant medical events and outcomes

If you use a minimalist approach to data collection and management, you can avoid the trap of *data mass*. Data mass is what happens when you spend lots of time and effort and money collecting information, making sure it's accurate, collating it all — then never interpreting and publishing it.

How to design a data sheet

I have found a very effective approach to data sheet design: gather four or five family practitioners and one disease area specialist and ask them to create your first draft. These people know the value of time and will create a data sheet that can be incorporated into, rather than imposed onto, their already busy schedules.

You know your design is good when physicians start using it in place of whatever existed before.

 You can hire trained data collectors or find existing staff to enter data. If you are working with physicians in other clinics, one office should act as a central data centre for quality assurance, consolidation, analysis and feedback.

 How people send in the information (fax, e-mail, hard copy) isn't important; be flexible. Your goal is to get as much information from as many people as possible, so make it easy for them.

Keeping people posted

When you measure health management and outcomes, you know whether your interventions are working, but unless you tell everyone else, they won't know if evidence-based management and health outcomes are improving.

All the people involved in the initiative will want feedback on the progress and results of the initiative. Develop a plan for communicating progress. For instance, newsletters sustain interest in a project that may run for several years.

You can read more about communication in Part IV.

Part IV

Healthy Communication

• •

In This Part

▶Educating patients

▶Reporting progress

▶Sharing experiences and knowledge

• •

*O*nce you've built the partnership and developed processes that work, producing demonstrably better management and outcomes, you're halfway there.

Remember, your experiences and achievements are valuable to others. To be a true centre of excellence in the patient health management world, you need to publish your results as widely and expeditiously as possible, so other people can adopt your best practices quickly.

Imagine one half of a centre of excellence as a castle of best practices — but a castle without a working drawbridge. True excellence comes only when the castle's expertise crosses the drawbridge to the community outside the knowledge centre. When you share information with other people, they'll know what interventions work best and can act on the knowledge.

In this part, I talk about the best ways to share information with patients and professionals. Let down that drawbridge!

Educating Patients

Education provides patients with information that helps them make the right care and lifestyle choices. Patients who take an active role in their health can improve their quality of life.

Knowledge can give patients hope. And hope can help patients deal with a disease that steals their happiness as it limits their ability to function.

We don't know the best way for health care professionals to educate patients about their treatment and their disease, since the subject hasn't been closely studied, but we do know that education is undeniably important.

We're still in the early days of developing educational programs for patients. We need to take more practical measures in the field of patient adherence to therapies, including:

- ✔ Better education for patients on the value of adherence and the risk of non-adherence

- ✔ Making measurement and feedback of patient adherence a regular part of disease management programs

Education means communication. Your goal should be two-way communication — patient-to-physician and patient-to-patient (and patient-to-family). When patients learn and communicate with each other and with their health care providers, their sense of well-being improves and the need for hospitalization decreases.

Better together

The effects of various education interventions haven't been studied closely, but, thanks to the CURATA project in Quebec, we do know that two education techniques have proven effective when used together:

- ✔ Evidence-based treatment algorithm, or recommended treatment for anticipated clinical situations

- ✔ Interactive workshops with physicians, specialists and patients

The CURATA project studied the effectiveness of these two educational interventions. Physicians monitored how patients with osteoarthritis, given medication instructions in two ways, used anti-inflammatory agents. They discovered that the algorithm helped teach patients how to comply with their treatment, but not as much as the interactive workshops. A combination of the two had the greatest effect in increasing compliance.

Kinds of education materials

You can offer your patients a range of health education materials to help explain disease and treatment options. Common materials include

- *Package inserts,* which include information about medications for patients written in easy-to-understand language from the pharmaceutical manufacturers
- Easy-to-read pamphlets
- Newsletters that explain disease and treatment options

Talking to health care providers is also important for your patients. The Web is another source of information, although you should provide a list of preferred Web sites with trusted content.

Contact patient groups like the Heart and Stroke Foundation or the Osteoporosis Society to discover what patient health education materials they publish. These materials can help you explain complex medical concepts to your patients.

Patient-to-patient communication

Invite patients to regular steering committee meetings and encourage them to share knowledge (for more about steering committee meetings, see Part II).

The ICONS patient health management initiative (see Part I) created Patient Education Days to foster patient-to-patient information exchanges. Organizers set up video teleconferences, regular steering committee meetings and special meetings with patient advocacy groups like the Heart and Stroke Foundation.

Spreading the Word

If you want your patient health management initiative to be successful, keep the channels of communication buzzing with information to and from all participants. Keep everyone in the loop and aware of progress. You'll also want to tell people outside your initiative how it's faring; after all, things won't get better if we keep our successes (and our problems) to ourselves.

Sharing information with participants

When you report the progress of your patient health management initiative, you show participants how their participation helps improve care. You're also nurturing their sense of civic responsibility, encouraging them to do their part because the task is important.

I've found that newsletters and meetings are great ways to keep people posted.

Hope in Alberta

Patients with heart failure are often very ill. Their many symptoms limit their ability to function at a level they associate with happiness or fulfillment. During the late 1980s and early 1990s, I was a physician at the Heart Function Clinic in Alberta. The clinic set up patient management processes and used evidence-based medical therapy to improve patients' longevity and quality of life.

Caring was very visible in this communication-rich outpatient setting. Hospitalizations decreased, and patients became more functional.

In the mid 1990s, the Heart Function Clinic asked patients to describe how they perceived their health. Not surprisingly, perceptions of quality of life improved with participation in the clinic. As well, patients expected continuing improvement — even patients with a progressive disease. Patients valued the information they received from physicians most of all.

Knowledge gives patients hope. The clinic developed user-friendly booklets with explanations that described symptoms and signs of a failing heart and provided information on treatments, including benefits and side effects. The clinic also encouraged physicians to smile when entering the patients' rooms and to ask patients about symptoms and treatment.

Newsletters and e-mails

Newsletters and e-mails can include information like

- ✔ Research highlights
- ✔ Statistics about patients, physicians, pharmacists and other people involved in the initiative
- ✔ Active lifestyle suggestions, reminders and tips
- ✔ Recipes for a healthier diet
- ✔ Important results from the initiative
- ✔ Spotlight on health care professionals on the team
- ✔ Answers to questions
- ✔ List of community resources

For a good example of a patient health management newsletter, visit the ICONS project at www.icons.ns.ca.

Your newsletter can be printed or electronic. An electronic newsletter or plain-text e-mail message is much less costly than a printed document.

Meetings

To maintain your partnerships and implement your various projects, schedule regular meetings. The meetings have two functions:

- ✔ **Reporting the status of research projects and interventions in progress:** Include feedback on patient recruitment, practices and outcomes and any issues or concerns with project progress.
- ✔ **Presentations by leading investigators and speakers:** Topics of interest to participants are ideal.

Try to balance feedback and edge-of-the-envelope education. Most people who come to the meetings will find the combination compellingly attractive. In your meetings, try to serve and stimulate the interests of those who attend.

You might try a modest social event before the business portion of the meeting. Socializing often encourages focus.

Keeping your peers posted

Communicating practice and outcome measurements is invaluable — I can't stress that enough. Communication helps generate interest and stimulate the innovative thoughts and ideas to make things better.

You might sometimes find it nerve-racking to measure, compare and communicate your group's practices and outcomes, but it can be managed in a collegial and anonymous, non-threatening manner. Feedback of actual practices is a major benefit of any patient health management project. Remember, a principal stimulus to do something different or to make something better is lost without feedback about less-than-optimal practices.

Two main ways to share your findings are

- ✔ The usual academic avenues of publications and presentations

- ✔ Outreach professional development programs that show physicians and nurses from other communities or medical practices how your patient health management initiative is operating

Financial incentives are not a silver bullet

Incentives are usually financial; for example, paying health care providers or patients when they adhere to best-practice guidelines in prescribing and taking their medicine. Incentives work, but they're not a silver bullet. They do not cure every care gap.

I have noticed a confused standard regarding the concept of financial incentives in health care. Is it acceptable for some people to make profits selling prescription drugs across international borders? Does it matter if the incentive is provided by a public or private payer? I have found no consensus on financial incentives in improving health care in Canada.

Incentives carry too much baggage and distract people from measurement, education and achievement. So, at least until the public debate on financing enters the next frank stage, I think we will be better served by avoiding any new and direct financial incentives to improve practices in patient health management programs.

Part V

More than Ten Patient Health Management Initiatives

• •

*T*he ICONS program (which I discuss in Part I) is, to date, the most important large-scale patient health management program in Canada. But there have been others. Programs that have demonstrated the effectiveness of community-based initiatives include:

AIMS

Alberta Improvements for Musculoskeletal Disorders Study was designed to establish the burden of illness for musculoskeletal diseases in the province and improve the appropriate use of health care resources for patients with acute and chronic musculoskeletal diseases in Alberta. (www.singlepoint.ca/clients/aims)

ASTHMA

The Alberta Strategy to Help Manage Asthma is a patient health management partnership composed of approximately 180 community physicians from across the province. The study also includes academic specialists in respiratory disease from the universities. The project is currently implementing interventions to close the care gaps it identified.

CANOAR

The primary goal of the Canadian Osteoarthritis Treatment Program was to identify the contemporary prescribing practices of a selected cohort of busy Ontario community care physicians. A secondary goal was to assess if reimbursement status influenced physician prescribing patterns.

COIN

A precursor of ICONS, the Clinical Quality Improvement Network was a partnership of physicians, nurses, pharmacists and other professional health stakeholders from community and university hospitals across Canada. Its goal was better management practices for the major cardiac diseases and a corresponding improvement in survival and quality of life for affected individuals.

CURATA

Concertation pour une utilisation raisonnée des anti-inflammatoires dans le traitement de l'arthrose was created in Quebec to evaluate two educational interventions on the appropriate use of anti-inflammatory agents in patients with osteoarthritis (see the "Better together" sidebar in Part IV for more information about CURATA).

Diabetes Hamilton

This public health intervention program was designed to improve the diabetes-related health of people with diabetes in the Hamilton region.

FORCE

The Falls, Fracture and Osteoporosis Risk Control and Evaluation project is a coalition of community, government and industry partners working to reduce osteoporosis-related complications in Northern Ontario. The project is centered in Sault Ste. Marie.

FTOP

Fracture? Think Osteoporosis! is a community-wide chronic disease management program for osteoporosis and its consequent fractures in the Hamilton-Wentworth Region. The goal is to improve diagnosis and treatment of osteoporosis in patients with fragility fractures and to decrease the rate of fractures in people older than 50 who have already had a fracture.

MAAUI

The Manitoba Anti-inflammatory Appropriate Utilization Initiative was designed to determine prescribing patterns for chronic anti-inflammatory drug use across the province, irrespective of disease diagnosis. The study identified care gaps. Intervention phases will close the gaps.

MOMM

The object of Maximizing Osteoporosis Management in Manitoba is to determine the prevalence of women with osteoporosis who are at increased risk for fracture and to study the care they receive. The goal is to anticipate care gaps and improve the use of evidence-based prevention and treatment strategies by using targeted interventions, by assessing changes in practice after intervention(s), and by assessing the impact of MOMM on disease awareness, patient diagnosis and treatment patterns.

ROCQ

Recognizing Osteoporosis and its Consequences in Quebec includes academic and community physicians from across the province. The project is multi-phased and projected to continue over several years.

TEAM

Known in French as VESPA, Towards Excellence in Asthma Management is a broad-based, patient health management partnership to improve asthma management in Quebec.

Part VI

The Ten Major Themes in Patient Health Management

• •

*P*atient health management initiatives have shown many more similarities than differences in clinical practice patterns and care gaps, irrespective of specific disease state, geography or physician type. In successful patient health management initiatives, some major themes inevitably recur, and in this part I describe the top ten.

Things can be better

Optimism is part of human nature. In fact, that things can be better seems obvious in light of the improvements in care since the early 1990s. There are still large care gaps in many of society's most burdensome illnesses. Things can always be better.

Care gaps are everywhere

We haven't closed the care gap entirely on any disease or medical condition.

Lately, problems we once thought were gone forever have returned. For instance, recent research shows that children in Canada are at risk of developing rickets — a bone disease that most Canadian physicians have not had to face for a generation. Vitamin D prevents the disease. But changing diets and habits (less time outside in the vitamin-D-producing sun) have reduced vitamin D levels in our bodies.

The re-emergence of old diseases shows that our work is never done. There are always new care gaps to close and old ones to keep closed.

Commitment to intervene is the cornerstone of success

Beware of the drowning sensation that comes from seeing so many opportunities and thinking you have too few resources to take advantage of them all.

Don't let your inability to do *everything* stop you from doing *something*. Choose one opportunity and make a commitment.

In patient health management, commitment is a two-fold virtue because there are two levels of commitment:

- ✔ **Level 1:** The commitment to act or intervene so you can make things better in practices and outcomes.

- ✔ **Level 2:** The commitment to take action that could result in significant and sustainable changes in practices and outcomes for patients. This means reaching out to community-based partners for help in finding and fixing care gaps.

Community-based partnerships are central

Your patient health management initiative needs community-based stakeholders as partners. Patients listen to members of their community and will participate if encouraged to do so. But community partners also are an untapped resource.

One of the most profound memories I carry is the sense of empowerment that developed among the patient participants in the ICONS patient health management initiative, particularly those that served on the steering committee.

These patients were probably more comfortable speaking on medical matters than most. I think they believed they had a responsibility to speak out on health policy matters in their town and province. The compulsion to enter the health debate was driven by their sense of involvement. They became confident they could contribute to the governance of a significant health initiative.

Measurement and communication are key processes

Effective patient health management requires an accurate snapshot of what the health teams are doing, a way to interpret that snapshot, and a method for disseminating the information to physicians. Measuring results and communicating them are crucial to improving outcomes.

Hope is a powerful facilitator for better care and outcomes

I think the belief that things can and will be better is an undervalued factor in health care management. It is not a new thing, and it does not often get mentioned in glossaries of evidence-based care. But hope is a powerful factor in patients' satisfaction with care and outcomes, particularly quality of life.

Perhaps there is some way to assess the power of hope. This will require more evidence. The insights that I developed on the value of hope in improving patients' perception of quality of life came from patient satisfaction surveys.

We do not ask patients about our daily practices often enough. We are probably missing valuable insights from patients, particularly as patients are increasingly educated in matters of disease and its treatment. I have come to think of the patient satisfaction survey as a regular opportunity to improve concordance between providers and patients about many issues in health care, sort of an extension of the value of concordance in improving patient compliance with prescriptions. Perhaps it would be possible to increase patient surveys, if tools can be developed. It is something worth pursuing.

Improving care is an enabler – a call to arms for all stakeholders

If there is one thing in health care that both provides gratification and acts as a driver to do even more and to do it better, it is seeing improvements in care and outcomes. Visible improvement works for both patients and providers as they make their complementary contributions to care.

Anyone can do it

It is a truism, but it is definitely true: the improvement of an important outcome, such as survival, is a result of a patient receiving prescriptions for the drugs that reduce risk. To achieve this end point we rely on physicians to prescribe the right drugs and we rely on patients to take them.

Improvement of other important outcomes, such as the need for re-hospitalization, may be determined by non-therapeutic factors, such as:

- The knowledge transferred to the patient, and what the patient accepts
- What the patient's family thinks and says
- The patient's level of income, age or setting

Many stakeholders can contribute to improved health outcomes. And they can contribute anywhere and in any disease state. It is not rocket science. It is commitment.

Include rather than isolate

In any area of endeavour there are many different ways to categorize people and processes. One of my colleagues believes there are two kinds of people at meetings: cooperators and competitors. I think of people as isolators or combiners, or in simpler language, splitters versus lumpers.

Splitters tend to break concepts and problems into many smaller parts and keep them there. Lumpers tend to group issues and problems and to seek partnership and integrated solutions. They take pride and comfort in an integrated approach and welcome the contributions of others.

In the area of compliance — patients taking their medications — splitters might assign responsibility exclusively to patients. Lumpers would say a number of players are responsible and any plan to fix things must include patients, doctors, pharmacists, nurses, dietitians — in other words, everyone.

In the design and governance of a patient health project, splitters might be inclined to keep all decision making within a small, expert group. Lumpers would involve as many people as possible early on, then work to make sure everyone can contribute.

The traditional solo physician practice is closer to the splitting concept; group practice and multidisciplinary care are closer to the lumping concept. My prediction is that as we acquire more knowledge and skills, the lumping of our expertise will be increasingly valued.

Health care providers who are best able to regroup our health workers so they deliver the best care in a continuous and flexible manner will be the most appreciated and successful — at least as judged by patients. Lumping, sharing and communicating our talents and opportunities will go a long way to making things better.

Things will be better

That things will get better isn't a false hope. The health and wealth of the nation are better than ever before and they will continue to improve. If we acknowledge the link between health and wealth, we may be able to move forward faster.

If we can create an environment where patients and consumers ask for more easily available, innovative health services, we'll have improved health outcomes and established the Canadian health industry as an important player in our economy.

The economic improvement from gains in health will produce more wealth for more investments in health and in other parts of our economy. In simple contemporary terms, if we improve our health system, we'll generate more than enough money to replace our Sea King helicopters.

What's Next

Merck Frosst Canada has partnered with key health care stakeholders, including patients, health care professionals, government and other pharmaceutical companies, in the search for better ways of managing the country's scarce health care resources and thereby helping to safeguard one of the world's most accessible and effective health care systems.

For assistance and information, contact us at info@terrymontague.ca or 1-800-567-2594.